DIET COOKBOOK FOR IBS

IRRITABLE BOWEL SYNDROME DIET RECOMMENDATIONS AND DIET PLAN

DR. KYLE PHELAN

Table of Contents

CHAPTER ONE

DIET FOR IBS

Irritable Bowel Syndrome Diet Recommendations

Finding and avoiding the foods that cause irritable bowel syndrome (IBS) symptoms is a major challenge for people with IBS.

Due to individual differences, there is no universally applicable diet plan. Irritable bowel syndrome (IBS) comes in a variety of forms, and the triggers that bring on symptoms in one person may be different from those that bring on symptoms in another (IBD-C).

While there is no one diet that helps everyone with IBS, there do seem to be a few that seem to work for different types of the disorder. Some might need modification to provide long-term relief, but with time and experimentation, you'll find the diet that works best for you and your IBS symptoms.

Benefits

The intestinal lining is not damaged in the medical condition known as irritable bowel syndrome, which is characterized by abdominal pain and alterations in bowel movement. Alternating bouts of diarrhea and constipation characterize mixed-type irritable bowel syndrome (IBS-M), a subtype of irritable bowel syndrome (IBS).

In the same way that the cause of IBS is unclear, there has been limited clinical research to evaluate the effectiveness of various diets in treating the disease. Scientists now know that certain foods and dietary practices are strongly linked to the emergence of IBS symptoms1.

The American College of Gastroenterology (ACG) published dietary guidelines in 2014 to help people with IBS better manage their symptoms.2 Of the dozens of diets reviewed by the ACG, only two were found to be significantly effective in treating IBS symptoms: the low-FODMAP diet and the gluten-free diet.

"Sensitivity to gluten is one of the most commonly reported reactions to food by patients with IBS," the ACG stated in 2021 guidelines, adding that a limited trial of the low-FODMAP diet was recommended to improve overall IBS symptoms3.

However, there is limited proof that these diets are effective for people with IBS or that they deal with the underlying causes of the disease, such as abnormal gut motility, heightened pain sensitivity, and an overgrowth of bacteria in the small intestine (SIBO).

It is recommended that a patient see a gastroenterologist for guidance as they work with a dietitian to develop a diet plan that is both effective and sustainable. Possible strategies include an elimination diet, in which IBS-suspected foods are eliminated from the diet and then reintroduced one at a time until symptoms return.

Details of Operation

Due to the multifaceted nature of IBS, there is no single best approach to diet planning. A two-step process is typically recommended by medical professionals:

Maintaining a regular eating schedule and minimizing intake of insoluble fiber, alcohol, caffeine, spicy foods, and fat are common first-line recommendations. It's also important to stay active on a regular basis and drink plenty of water.

If these treatments don't help, your doctor may recommend trying a gluten-free or low-FODMAP diet.

If changes are insufficient or inconsistent, further tweaking may be required. In most cases, this means learning to recognize and avoid the foods that set off an individual's immune system, whether due to an allergy or intolerance. To make sure you're getting the nutrients you need each day, you may want to consult a dietitian or nutritionist.

List of Foods Known to Trigger Irritable Bowel Syndrome

A Diet Low in Fermentable Short Chain Carbohydrates

An abbreviation for fermentable oligo-, disaccharides-, mono-, and polyols. These are the common short-chain carbohydrates that cause an increase in liquid and gas volume during digestion in the small and large intestine.

The symptoms of irritable bowel syndrome (IBS) include gas, bloating, and abdominal pain, all of which can be triggered by eating too many foods high in fermentable oligosaccharides, sugars, and proteins (FODMAPs). Therefore, it stands to reason that avoiding foods high in FODMAPs can help prevent and/or alleviate these symptoms. Numerous commonly consumed foods are high in FODMAPs, making diet planning difficult.

Five distinct FODMAP classes include:

Fruit sugars (found in wheat, onions, garlic, barley, cabbage, and broccoli)

"• Fructose" (found in fruit, honey, and high-fructose corn syrup)

Specific Galactooligosaccharides (found in legumes and beans)

• Lactose (found in milk and other dairy foods)

• Polyols (found in stone fruits, sweet potatoes, apples, and celery)

As part of an elimination diet, a low-FODMAP diet is structured in two phases:5

FODMAP-heavy foods are avoided during this phase for a limited time, typically between three and six weeks.

Phase 2 involves reintroducing the eliminated foods back into the diet one FODMAP type at a time to determine how well they are tolerated.

The American Gastroenterological Association (AGC) suggests doing so with the help of a qualified gastrointestinal nutritionist. In the event that this is not possible, they recommend that you request high-quality materials from your healthcare provider to help you through the process in a responsible manner.3

With proper execution, response rates in the hundreds per hour range are possible. A recent study by Monash University found that approximately 75% of people with IBS who tried a low-FODMAP diet experienced significant symptom relief.

Eat No Gluten!

Gluten is a protein found in foods containing cereal grains like wheat, rye, and barley, and many people with IBS report an improvement in symptoms when they eliminate gluten from their diet even if they do not have celiac disease.[6]

It is debatable whether or not gluten contributes to irritable bowel syndrome. Some researchers believe that irritable bowel syndrome (IBS) is a form of non-celiac gluten sensitivity, a disorder similar to celiac in which gluten triggers adverse gastrointestinal symptoms.[7] However, there are also researchers who believe that fructan, a type of FODMAP, is to blame for IBS rather than gluten.

If the low-FODMAP diet doesn't help, going gluten-free may be tried. The amount of gluten you eat may be gradually increased to determine if you have a safe tolerance range for the protein if they do. Doing so might free you from having to adhere to such stringent dietary restrictions and open up a whole new world of delicious foods.

Consuming less than 20 ppm of gluten per day is considered to be gluten-free. Gluten levels below 100 ppm are considered safe for those with celiac disease.

Serological testing for celiac disease, including

Transglutaminase IgA antibody and total IgA levels, should precede the initiation of a gluten-free diet. If patients have low IgA levels (approx 2-3% of the population) then the Deamidated gliadin peptide IgG antibody is used for screening. If the serological tests are equivocal, then genetic testing is the next step.

Your doctor may test you for food allergies or intolerances if your symptoms persist despite following a gluten-free or low-FODMAP diet. For this reason, testing and consultation with an allergist may be necessary. Your diet, then, would need to be further adjusted accordingly.

CHAPTER TWO

Can Sugar Intolerance Cause Irritable Bowel Syndrome?

Regardless of the diet plan you choose, consistency is essential. Irritable bowel syndrome (IBS) diets are long-term plans that may call for major adjustments to your current way of eating and living. This may involve regular exercise for weight loss and normalizing bowel function in addition to avoiding alcoholic beverages, caffeine, and fatty foods. If you're not active and/or overweight, a change in diet may not be enough to alleviate your irritable bowel syndrome symptoms.

There is no evidence to support the "as needed" use of a low-FODMAP diet or gluten-free diet for the short-term relief of acute symptoms. In this regard, it may be helpful to increase the consumption of prunes and bran on days when constipation symptoms are severe, or to increase the consumption of water if you have diarrhea.

What to Eat for IBS-C

Constipation is a common symptom of irritable bowel syndrome, and increasing your fiber intake can help. It's best to gradually up your dosage to give your body time to adjust. As a rule of thumb, soluble fiber is better tolerated by people with IBS than insoluble fiber is.10

In addition, you should prioritize eating foods high in healthy fats like polyunsaturated and monounsaturated oils. High-saturated-fat and high-sugar foods are well-known culprits in causing digestive issues like constipation.

Foods That Are IBS-C-Approved

Cereals and breads made with whole grains

Bran from oats

- Produce (especially apples, pears, kiwifruit, figs, and kiwifruit)

- Produce (especially green leafy vegetables, sweet potato, and Brussels sprouts)

- Legumes, such as beans and peas

The use of dried fruit

The Drink: Juice from Prunes

Fat-free milk (in moderation)

Kefir and Yogurt

Chicken without the skin

• Fish (especially fatty fish like salmon and tuna)

• Seeds (especially chia seed and ground flaxseed)

Thin soups

Foods That Don't Fit the IBS-C Diet

Simple carbohydrates like white bread, pasta, and crackers

Green bananas

• Persimmons

- Fried or quick meals

baked goods (cookies, muffins, cakes)

Plain rice

Butter and other dairy products with a high fat content (including ice cream)

Intoxicants: Alcohol (especially beer)

The Meat We Eat • Beef

Toasted potato chips

- Chocolate

* Rich, velvety soups

Dietary Recommendations for Irritable Bowel Syndrome/Disease Crohn's

Staying with bland foods is recommended if your IBS symptoms include diarrhea. Avoiding foods that are fatty, greasy, or creamy is recommended because they can stimulate intestinal contractions and lead to cramping and diarrhea.

Stay away from insoluble fiber, as it causes diarrhea by attracting and absorbing water in the digestive tract. Though you should try to eat plenty of fruits and vegetables, you should keep your fiber intake to less than 1.5 grams per half-cup during acute episodes1.

Foods Acceptable for Individuals with Irritable Bowel Syndrome

Simple carbohydrates like white bread, pasta, and crackers

Complete grains (unless you are gluten intolerant)

Plain rice

• Oatmeal

Chicken without the skin

Protein sources that are low in saturated fats, such as lean meat

- Skinny fish (like halibut, flounder, and cod)

- Eggs

- Potatoes, steamed, boiled, or baked

Legumes, such as beans and peas,

- Bananas

You can drink rice milk, almond milk, or coconut milk.

- Lactose-free, low-fat milk

Yogurt with probiotic cultures that is low in fat (in moderation)

- 100% pure, unsweetened fruit juice

Examples: • Rigid Cheeses (in moderation)

- Applesauce

- Tofu

Foods That Aren't OK for People with Irritable Bowel Syndrome, Type D

- Fried or quick meals

Sweetened foods (e.g., baked goods)

Foods high in saturated fats, such as: (e.g., bacon and sausage)

Items that have been processed and then re-cooked (e.g., hot dogs and lunchmeat)

Foods like sardines and other canned fish in oil

Vegetables with a cruciform shape (e.g., cauliflower, broccoli, cabbage, and Brussels sprouts)

Eat more raw vegetables and salads.

Foods containing legumes (like beans and peas)

* Citrus Fruits

• Caffeine

• Dairy products, including milk (e.g., butter and soft cheeses)

Carbonated beverages

Sweetened fruit juices and nectars

• Alcohol

Fruits that have been dried and packaged

• Miso

Synthetic sugar substitutes (sorbitol and xylitol)

Time Frame Recommendation

Smaller, more frequent meals are easier on the digestive system than three large ones, which is why they are recommended for many people with IBS. This prevents the bowels from becoming full suddenly and then empty for five or six hours straight, promoting regular, gentle bowel movements.

On the other hand, some people with IBS-D are told to eat a large breakfast or drink coffee first thing in the morning to encourage bowel movement (referred to as a gastrocolic reflex). Keeping to your regular routine in the morning could help you avoid accidents all day. It also helps to sit up straight during meals instead of slouching on the couch, and to go for a short walk after eating.

One of the factors in whether or not you experience symptoms of irritable bowel syndrome is your diet. By pausing purposefully between bites and eating more slowly, you can cut down on the amount of air you take in while you eat.

Eating quickly, drinking from a straw, or chewing gum all increase the likelihood of experiencing gas, bloating, and abdominal pain because they all involve swallowing air.

CHAPTER THREE

Advice on the Kitchen

First and foremost, those on an IBS diet should stay away from anything deep-fried. No matter which form of IBS you have, you can forget about eating your favorite fried foods like French fries, donuts, and fried chicken.

Instead, use very little oil when grilling, roasting, or frying meats. Instead of adding oil to the pan, you can spray it directly onto the meat for a healthier and more efficient cooking method. Lightly searing meat, chicken, or fish to get a nice crust and then finishing it in a hot 425°F oven for a few minutes is a restaurant-quality method. Also, maybe think about getting an air fryer.

Vegetables

Vegetables are easier to digest after being steamed, which is particularly helpful for people who suffer from diarrhea. If raw salads are too much for your stomach, try one of the many delicious cooked salad variations (like a Mediterranean Heart of Palm Salad or a Grilled Eggplant Salad). Vegetables, tomatoes, and fruit are all easier to digest after being peeled.

Use a squeeze of lemon or lime, some chopped fresh herbs, or a mild salsa made from tomatoes or mangoes in place of salad dressings or sauces.

Beans

Canned beans may cause gas, but you can minimize its effects by rinsing and soaking them in cold water for 30 minutes before eating them. Beans should be soaked in hot water for a few hours, then in cold water overnight if you're making them from scratch, before being cooked slowly in fresh water until very soft.

There is an opinion that cooking beans with ground ajwain (a type of caraway) or epazote (a Mexican herb with a pine-like aroma) can significantly reduce their gassiness. The lack of evidence does not preclude testing the theory.

Modifications

Diets low in fermentable oligosaccharides and polyols (FODMAPs) and gluten are both thought to be safe for adults, provided that the DRIs for protein, carbohydrates, and nutrients are met. However, because these diets typically exclude whole grains, dairy, and other vital nutrients, nutritional deficiencies are common.

During pregnancy, when nutritional needs are at their peak, these worries only grow in intensity. For instance, it's common knowledge that those who follow a gluten-free diet consume less of these nutrients:

- Iron

- Folate

- Fiber

- Calcium

- Thiamine

- Riboflavin

- Niacin

There is no way to have a healthy pregnancy without all of those nutrients. Although prenatal vitamins can help make up for this, it still shows how dangerous these diets can be if not closely monitored.

For this and other reasons, children, who require a healthy, balanced diet to ensure normal growth and development, should approach low-FODMAP and gluten-free diets with extreme caution.

When a child has been diagnosed with IBS and has not shown improvement with more conservative treatments, their doctor may recommend a low-FODMAP diet. A gluten-free diet is also only appropriate for kids who have been medically confirmed to have celiac disease or non-celiac gluten intolerance.

Dietary supplementation is commonly recommended to help improve nutrition, and it is best to follow a diet under the supervision of a healthcare provider or registered dietitian.

Considerations

Low-FODMAP and gluten-free diets are two examples of extremely restrictive eating plans that may be challenging to maintain. It will take effort on your part and support from loved ones for these to be successful. You can overcome the hardships of the diet and start to manage your IBS by keeping your mind on the positive effects it will have on your health and well-being rather than on the foods you can't have.

Status of General Health

There are good points and drawbacks to both the low-FODMAP and gluten-free diets. Since many of the foods included in the diets are thought to be beneficial to diabetes and hypertension (high blood pressure), their use is generally safe for those with these conditions.

Both diets have a learning curve, and some people experience temporary discomforts like fatigue and gas during that time. Most of these go away by themselves, though some (like food cravings) require effort to manage.

What really matters is how these diets will affect your health in the long run. Some scientists are concerned that these kinds of restrictive diets (especially when used for reasons other than medical necessity) can lead to disordered eating, as evidenced in part by a 2017 study from Sweden that found young girls with celiac disease were 4.5 times more likely to have anorexia than those without the disorder.

There is evidence that restricting certain foods can affect heart health, and some worry that using such diets for an extended period of time could permanently alter the gut flora, thereby increasing the risk of bowel infection.11

Without the protective whole grains, the risk of cardiovascular disease is increased, according to a study published in 2017 in the journal BMJ Clinical Research.12

Environmental compatibility and real-world applicability

The restriction of foods that are high in fermentable oligosaccharides and short chain carbohydrates (FODMAPs) and gluten can be isolating, which can be a drawback of these diets. According to a review of studies published in 2018 in

Gastroenterology & Hepatology,13 the persistent dedication to a restricted diet contributes to increased rates of social isolation as well as feelings of anxiety and inadequacy if adherence to the diet falls short. Fortunately, there are ways to mitigate some of these concerns.

Consuming in a Restaurant

In contrast to earlier decades, nowadays there are many more restaurants that cater to those who need to avoid gluten when dining out. Even fast-food and casual-dining franchises have joined in.

You can still find something to eat at most restaurants, even if they don't offer gluten-free or low-FODMAP options, by looking at their online menu ahead of time. If you call ahead of time and let the restaurant know about your dietary restrictions, they may be able to make some adjustments.

Readying of Food

For people with IBS, the ability to control what goes into their food when cooking at home is invaluable. The popularity of low-FODMAP and gluten-free diets has prompted many food bloggers to share their tried-and-true recipes online.

There is an increasing number of gluten-free meal kit delivery services, and a few of them have begun to offer low-FODMAP options, which is great news for those who are too busy to shop for and prepare their own meals.

Cost

The high price of gluten-free and low-FODMAP foods in supermarkets is another problem.

The cost of eating gluten-free can be prohibitive, as a 2018 study in the United Kingdom found that gluten-free foods were 159% more expensive than their regular counterparts.14 (although the costs can usually be reduced by avoiding packaged foods and eating real foods prepared at home).

However, snacks, spices, dressings, and soup bases that are low in FODMAPs are only available from a small number of specialty producers, including Rachel Pauls Food and Fody. These are typically quite pricey as well.

The Downside

Adverse reactions to low-FODMAP and gluten-free diets are common, but many of them go away as your body adjusts to the new eating routine.

CHAPTER FOUR

There was a significant increase in weight.

Sensation of Urgent Need to Detoxify the Bowel

• Fatigue

Chapped lips

Regular urination is a symptom of.

Consequences of a Gluten-Free Diet

- Headaches

- Nausea

- Fatigue

- Constipation

Increased hunger

There was a significant increase in weight.

- Difficulty focusing

Pain in the legs

Though these side effects may be unpleasant, they are usually seen as a fair price to pay by those who turn to an IBS diet in the face of debilitating symptoms.

Having a Community Behind You and Offering Help

Starting an IBS diet on your own can be a daunting task. If you try to keep your loved ones in the dark about your decision, you may find it more difficult to deal with the emotional fallout.

Get them involved by explaining IBS and how the diet will help. It may pave the way for you to make dietary changes that benefit your whole family, rather than just yourself. By involving them, you increase the odds that they will support the diet and decrease the chances that they will try to derail it by calling it a fad.

Notifying your doctor of any difficulties you're having with the diet will allow them to make necessary adjustments. You should also try to find people who have been through something similar and can relate to what you're going through.

Facebook is full of groups dedicated to helping people with IBS, and the nonprofit IBS Patient Support Group also hosts online forums for discussion and support. Your doctor may also be aware of local in-person resources for those dealing with IBS.

If you find yourself in need of some extra motivation, encouragement, or inspiration, there are even low-FODMAP apps and gluten-free apps to download.

Comparing the Low-FODMAP and Elemental Diets

There is an overgrowth of bacteria in the small intestine, a condition known as small intestinal bacterial overgrowth (SIBO). As such, a low-FODMAP diet is often used to treat IBS, as it is one of the most common contributing factors.

Recent years, however, have seen the development of a disease-specific elemental diet designed to impede bacterial growth and restore normal gut flora in people with SIBO.

The prolonged use of fluids containing primarily amino acids, sugars, vitamins, and minerals is at the heart of the controversy surrounding this liquid diet. Due to the potential for hypersensitivity in some individuals, it is typically protein-free or contains only trace amounts of protein. As a rule, fat consumption should make up no more than 1% of daily calories.

CHAPTER FIVE

Potential Rewards and Potential Risks

Evidence suggests that the elemental diet can aid those undergoing antibiotic treatment for SIBO. The diet is effective because it supplies the first portion of the small intestine with food. Few nutrients are available to "feed" the gut bacteria by the time the liquid reaches the lower bowel. This mechanism of action has the potential to aid in reducing bacterial proliferation.

After 14 days on the elemental diet, 74 of 93 adults had improved symptoms of irritable bowel syndrome (IBS), and this number increased to 79 by day 21 of the study.15 However, other studies have not found similar results.

The prolonged restriction of protein and fat is a second major difficulty of the elemental diet, after maintaining the diet itself. Fat and protein deprivation can cause a wide variety of negative health effects, including weakness, fatigue, loss of muscle mass, irregular heartbeat, infection, and more.

A Diet Low in Fermentable Short Chain Carbohydrates

For the long-term management of IBS symptoms

Ability to be put to continuous use

Has the ability to manage itself

You can buy groceries at any supermarket.

• Adverse effects are usually not severe

• It can be hard to stick to a routine.

Raw Food Diet

As a result of its stigma, it is typically only used as a last resort when all other strategies have been exhausted.

- Typically only used for a maximum of three weeks

- Must be monitored by a doctor or other medical professional

- You can get a powdered diet from your doctor or a health food store.

- Disabling side effects are common.

- It can be hard to stick to a routine.

A Word

Although there may be a complex interplay between what you eat and irritable bowel syndrome, you can take steps to improve your condition by altering both your eating habits and the foods you select. Conscious dietary planning can work in tandem with prescribed medication to help you manage the symptoms of irritable bowel syndrome.

REGULARLY INQUIRED ABOUT

For IBS, what kinds of foods should you avoid, and how?

Work with your doctor or a dietitian to ensure you're getting enough of the right nutrients if you plan on trying an elimination diet. They may advise you to keep a food diary to record how you feel before and after removing certain foods from your diet. In addition, they can advise you on the duration and specific foods to cut out of your diet.

To what kinds of foods should people with irritable bowel syndrome try to avoid?

Saturated fats, dairy products, high-FODMAP fruits and vegetables, beans, and artificial sweeteners are common food triggers for irritable bowel syndrome. Before cutting any foods out of your diet, talk to your doctor.